FROM THE INSIDE OUT

· ·

YOUR EASY to READ, MOTIVATIONAL GUIDE to NATURAL PATHWAYS USED in the FIGHT against PREMATURE AGING

STEPHANIE SCHIFF,
DC, DCN, F.A.C.A.C.N.

To my dear son, Spencer, and to anyone who has, in any way, however small, helped give me the confidence to develop this book. From my loving parents, to complete strangers who left comments on my blog, and everyone in between, thank you.

CONTENTS

INTRODUCTION

In the fight for longevity and the prevention of premature aging, we must first focus on the inside. There are numerous ways the beauty industry, not to mention the cosmetic—I mean, *medical*—industry can help your body beat the aging clock, and that's great. However, if we ignore the ways in which *internal* factors—such as lifestyle habits, what we eat, and the supplements we may or may not take—affect us, then all of those *external* measures some of us take to look and feel better or younger won't do much good in the long run. This book is about attaining and maintaining longevity.

I hope that by reading this book—which, let's face it, is short, so it won't take long—you'll be enlightened along your path to longevity (and by this I mean *living long*) and armed with the ammunition (I did not say it would be peaceful) to win the battle against premature aging and the debilitating diseases that come with it.

A good amount of nutritional reading material available today can be quite monotonous or intimidating. There is so much conflicting advice out there regarding nutrition. Some people would rather just ignore all of the different and endless "news" stories they come across. This is why I found it necessary to write this very easy-to-read, unintimidating book for you to use as a reference. This book is a short compilation of information regarding what I feel are some of the most important and basic health choices you can make to help keep you staying young and healthy. It should be painless to read, as if I'm just talking to you and not as if you're reading a boring nutritional textbook.

I want you to feel confident that you are getting some of the latest information at hand. At the very least, I hope you receive the motivation to put in a real effort and take action toward fighting off internal aging and seizing control of your health. Once you do that, you'll take control of your life. Read this book and have fun along your road to reversing, or at least slowing down, the clock.

CHAPTER 1

LIFESTYLE HABITS

Have you ever thought about what life will be like fifty years from now in terms of aging? With all of the biotechnological and medical advancements of the future (for example, stem cell research), will we be able to open up a "body-part storage account" and then, on an as-needed basis, waltz into our doctor's office (which happens to have an endless supply of replacement body parts growing inside glowing containers) and request a new replacement part? Maybe even a new head? What about keeping your head and receiving a whole new body? This could all be possible in the future. Yes, bioengineering technology, or whatever they call it, might enable us to have this kind of Frankenstein-humanoid service by the time you or I reach old age.

Well, I don't know about you, but I am not waiting that long, nor am I thrilled with the idea of having my body separated from my head in order to receive a new, young version of my body or vise versa. So I am, and have been for many years now, on a path paved with knowledge that includes healthy lifestyle choices, the right nutrients that promote preventative health care, and powerful bang-for-your-buck foods. I have chosen to cling to the will to fight the battle of premature aging and to do *most* of it (yes, I do cheat sometimes) naturally.

When you hear the words "anti-aging" and "longevity," do you think of the big picture and ask yourself, *Am I healthy? Am I living my life, for the most part, the right way to let myself live a long and healthy life?*

Did you really think about *every* way in which you live before you answered those questions? When most people hear the word "anti-aging," they think of what people in general, or they themselves, *look* like. They think only of the unfortunate external effects of aging, such as wrinkles and the graying of hair, these effects being the kind you can cheat Mother Nature a bit with great inventions such as hair coloring (I told you I cheat some). If this sounds familiar to you, I hope to soon change your way of thinking. No, you do not have to stop coloring your hair, getting chemical peels from your dermatologist, or stop whatever else you do to help yourself look and feel younger. You just have to add the more important elements to your battle.

Some of you may already be on the right track if you are focusing on eating right and taking the right nutritional supplements. While this is excellent, you must not, however, forget the most important area in the fight against premature aging and illness. This crucial area is your lifestyle habits. The first chapter in this book focuses on lifestyle habits because the *way* in which you live sets the *foundation* upon which you *build* a healthy lifestyle. Only after you adopt good habits while nixing the bad ones can you begin the process of healthy living and fight off premature aging and illness. You want to be able to get a good grasp on your plan of action. Remember, this is war.

Use the information in this book as your guide to forming your own personal modus operandi. I always say about everything, "You gotta have a plan." So enjoy this chapter and get serious about your health, then start your plan today.

Smoking—It's a Killer

By now most of the world's population knows that smoking isn't just bad for you; it will kill you. Smoking is the number-one reason both women and men die each year of lung cancer, heart disease, and stroke. If you smoke, don't even bother reading the rest of this book unless you commit to stop smoking now. You actually have a chance of reversing a lot of the damage done to your lungs if you stop smoking now, unless you are ninety-five and have been smoking two packs a day for the past seventy-five years. If so, then, well, good luck. Hopefully, for your sake, I was wrong about the whole Frankenstein thing and you can start growing your new lungs today. Gosh, I am sorry. I am really being insensitive. I will stop now. Thankfully, in the world we live in today, lung transplants are an option for some. Thank God.

A lot of people who smoke really do make a conscious effort to stop smoking, but they can't. They try over and over again. If you are one of those people, you still need to try and try again. Only this time try something new. For example, try to never be idle. Keep yourself busy. Don't sit down (oh...sorry...knitting is usually done sitting down). Take walks with others who have already quit and know what it is like to try to quit. Suck on sugar-free candy canes and lollipops. My friends from college did this, and supposedly it worked. Try nicotine patches, prescribed by your doctor, if you must. Work out at the gym. Get therapy. In other words, do whatever you need to do to quit, as long as it is healthy. (And last time I checked, replacing cigarettes with food is *not* healthy.) Ask your friends to tell you over and over again that you smell like an ashtray (because you do), and that might do the trick. Try everything until you succeed. *Just please stop smoking.*

Sleep

Guess what? All of the claims you have heard about the negative effects of not getting enough sleep are absolutely true. No matter how much you exercise, how well you eat, how many supplements you take, how many annual wellness exams you have, and whatever else you do to take good care of yourself, if you do not get seven to nine hours of sleep per night (children need more) on a regular basis, your immune system is in a constant state of compromise (danger).

It works like this: Your body uses your immune system to fight off everything from the common cold to major life-threatening illnesses and everything in between, including free radicals—which are one of the culprits in the aging process—and premature aging. When you don't get enough sleep, your body does not get the rest it needs in order for the immune system to take over during that rest period to do what it needs to do—fight. With inadequate amounts of sleep, you send your body into overdrive. You then make your immune system run uphill while being rundown, until eventually it breaks down and is unable to fight off anything. This is when you start to get chronic illnesses or at least feel chronically lousy. Your body then oxidizes at a faster rate because free radicals can *freely* take over. The free radicals are having a party inside your body because your immune system is not working actively to fight them off. Thus the internal aging process is greatly accelerated. Your skin, nails, hair, eyes, and metabolism (yes, with less sleep, you burn less fat) will suffer greatly, and you will be much more vulnerable to bacterial infections, viruses, and cancers.

All of the above does not happen with just one sleepless night. Everyone has those once in a while. These effects result from cumulative sleep loss over weeks, months, or, unfortunately for some, years. As hard as it might seem for some people who complain every day that they have too many things to do to worry about sleep, these people (are you one of them?) must still make getting seven to nine hours of sleep a priority. If you are one of these very busy people, you should, in fact, make getting eight to ten hours of sleep your priority. That way, if you aim for eight hours of sleep, you will most likely get seven. This is better than aiming for seven and getting six, right?

It should not matter how many kids you have, how many jobs you are working, or how many needy, lazy husbands you have. (Sorry, men. We women don't love you any less, but it's true. The majority of you are needy and lazy—just a fact.) If you are so busy that you can't get a good night's sleep on a regular basis, you are already prone to illness and premature aging due to sheer stress, which I touch upon in a later chapter. If this is you, lessen the load. Lose the husband already. I am just kidding of course. If you are lucky enough to have kids, a career, a lazy—I mean, *loving*—husband, and all this stuff and people around you to take care of, realize how important *you* are and how important it is to take care of *you*. After all, what would your family and career be like if you were no longer healthy enough to care for them?

To ensure a regular good night's sleep, you must work everything around your eight hours of sleep. That's right. It may sound crazy to you busy, busy people to put sleep first, but it's easy. First set yourself a bedtime (yes, just like you do for your kids). Go to sleep *at the same time* each night, except for Friday and Saturday nights. Make your weeknight bedtime at, let's say, ten p.m. You should have no problem waking up each morning at six a.m. without an alarm clock. That's right. If you need to wake up with an alarm clock, this simply means you are not getting enough sleep. Maybe you need ten hours. Get the sleep you need. Go to bed at an earlier time. Remember, work everything around your sleep. Only nursing mothers have an excuse not to.

Now back to the alarm clock. I will bet that you did not know that waking up to an alarm clock threatens your health. This is because instead of waking up naturally your alarm disrupts, with a shock, your internal, biological clock, your circadian rhythm. This disruption is slightly hard on your heart, especially if you have any sort of heart problem already. If you need an alarm to wake you up, you are not letting your natural sleep cycle finish, which also can compromise your immune system.

An interesting but scary fact is that each and every spring, on the morning after daylight savings when you lose an hour, your risk of having a heart attack increases by about 10 percent. Your biological clock gets totally thrown out of whack because of your having lost one hour of sleep. A heart attack because of one hour! This is an example of how much we need sleep and how important it is not to interrupt our natural circadian rhythm (sleep cycle).

Make it an absolute priority for you and your family members to get enough sleep every day. Good night.

The Power of Exercise

Exercise is an extremely important element in the battle against aging and maintaining the integrity of your health in general. Regular exercise is key to raising your metabolism, maintaining healthy lung and heart function, keeping oxygen flowing through your vessels, and fighting bone density loss. It also helps keep you mentally and emotionally healthy. Exercise has been proven to help regulate a person's sleeping patterns, boost the immune system, and immediately lift one's mood. Regular exercise keeps your confidence level higher, making you more socially active.

So get your butt off the couch! Get up and out and get physical. It doesn't matter what you choose to do—just do it.

There has been a lot of talk floating around regarding which type of exercise is best—for example walking versus running, weight-bearing versus non-weight bearing, etc. While weight-bearing exercise helps prevent bone density loss, if you worry too much about which type of exercise you need to do, you might leave out the kinds of activities you enjoy, thereby doing nothing at all. All you really need to know and remember is that whichever form of exercise you choose, do it regularly. Every day would be excellent, although daily exercise isn't realistic for most people. So just make sure that your exercise of choice includes brisk movement for at least thirty minutes at least three days per week. Every other day, which ends up being four days per week, is best. The schedule can go something like this: exercise on Monday, Wednesday, Friday, and Sunday. This schedule will allow your joints and muscles to rest between each day of exercise while you still get a healthy amount of exercise. It's also a good idea to stretch on the days when you do not exercise.

Again the most important factor when considering a form of exercise or activity is to choose something you enjoy. There are so many different kinds of activities that there is just no excuse not to exercise. Your exercise of choice can be swimming, walking, bicycling, dancing, martial arts, or whatever. Just have fun! Remember, engage in *brisk* activities. Activities such as knitting and bird watching are not forms of exercise. Some of you might hate me for this, but I do not consider yoga a form of brisk, heart-loving exercise. In other words the exercise must be aerobic. Yes, I have done yoga, and I respect it, but you can do yoga on your "off" days. Think of yoga as stretching. So get moving and go have some fun!

Whole-Mouth Health

Here is an interesting fact. Believe it or not, the way and frequency in which you clean your teeth and gums (actually, your entire mouth) profoundly affects your overall health. On a local level, there are the issues of stains, bad breath, cavities, gum disease, and the natural, progressive wearing down of tooth enamel. As you age, your teeth become more fragile and your gums more sensitive; your enamel wears down at a faster rate; and you must become even more diligent at whole-mouth (teeth, gums, and tongue) hygiene. Learn at an early age, which most of you do, the importance of teeth cleaning, and hopefully you will not have to succumb to those frightful things they call dentures. I don't know about you, but every time I see a commercial in which a set of those fake teeth with the attached pink rubber "gums" are dropped into a cup of fizzy blue cleaning liquid, I feel like sprinting to my dentist for an extra checkup and a cleaning. I do not want to have to wear those things.

I've covered the local level of the mouth itself, but there are, however, much more serious health risks associated with neglecting to properly take care of your mouth (remember, teeth, gums, *and* tongue). Just by regularly flossing twice a day you can considerably lower your chances of getting heart disease. It's true. A great deal of bacteria hides in the gum line between teeth. These bacteria can find ways into your bloodstream and then to your heart.

Poor dental hygiene can lead to other illnesses. Some studies suggest that you can significantly lower your risk of developing certain cancers by practicing good oral hygiene, which includes brushing, flossing, and tongue scraping (a huge amount of bacteria can be found at the back of the tongue). Don't forget to follow these steps with an oral antiseptic rinse that may or may not include fluoride. Do all of this, and do it twice per day, and you're good to go. Finally don't forget your semi-annual dental checkups.

The Importance of Annual Physicals

Speaking of checkups, you must get an annual wellness physical. This preventative form of care will ensure your doctor of the best chances of detecting any serious illness early, giving you the best opportunity to beat it. Take advantage, even at the extra cost if you can afford it, of available medical screening tests, specifically blood tests. A lot of people don't know about all of the available screening tests, and most doctors assume you don't want them because you won't want to pay out of pocket for them. Each year try to budget for the tests your insurance does not cover. These tests are worth it. Medical technology is advancing at a rapid rate while new screening tests for various diseases are introduced every year. A screening blood test for breast cancer should be out by 2013. Ask your doctor about any new tests every year.

The most common annual tests for women include blood pressure, mammogram, pelvic/pap, and a complete blood workup, which should include (but may not be covered by insurance) CA-125, ESR, and vitamin D levels. Other necessary tests are bone density, cholesterol, fasting blood sugar, a colon brush test, a whole-body skin check for precancerous/cancerous moles, and, after age forty-five to fifty (depending on family history), a colonoscopy.

The most common annual tests for men are blood pressure, a complete blood workup (including PSA, ESR, and vitamin D levels), a prostate exam, a colon brush test, cholesterol, fasting blood sugar, a whole-body skin check, and a colonoscopy after age forty-five to fifty.

There are many other tests your doctor may feel you need. The ones I listed are the basics. Again, ask for any available cutting-edge tests that may be applicable to you. Preventative medicine is the best medicine.

Also make sure you are honest with your doctor at every annual checkup. Discuss any unhealthy changes in your lifestyle. No matter how minor or embarrassing you think they are, your doctor needs to know about them.

Get a Chiropractor

You might think I am biased on the subject of chiropractors because I am a chiropractor. You are correct! Of course I have a positive view of chiropractors, and I am quite aware that not all people agree that chiropractors are necessary. I have heard all of the quackery jokes. The truth is there is no quackery involved when it comes to treating back pain due to injury, a herniated disc, or sciatica. The number-one reason for absences in the workplace is incapacitating neck and/or back pain. A chiropractor can successfully thwart the need for vertebral, spinal, or disc surgery. These surgeries are only 50 percent effective. Fortunately there are chiropractors. Chiropractors are the only doctors who focus on all of the joints in the body, especially the spine. The spine, or vertebrae, is the gateway *from* your nerves (which stem from your brain and spinal cord) *to all* of the muscles and organs in your body. These nerves—or your nervous system rather—control every other system in your body.

One trick to staying healthy is to periodically check in with your vertebral spine via a chiropractor, from the base of your head all the way down to your buttocks and also all of the other joints in your arms and legs. It is helpful to know about any neuro/nerve problems early on, before these problems become major by affecting organ systems or by causing other problems and pain in your neck and back. In the case of a herniated disc, most people wait until they practically have to crawl through the door of a chiropractor's office due to pain before they see a chiropractor, or worse, they first seek out a medical doctor for a prescription for painkillers while letting their problem exacerbate. The drugs are a temporary bandage, not a fix. The problem will continue to worsen until the patient requires surgery. Once the patient has had surgery, he or she will be even more incapacitated, need more drugs, and so on. Did I mention the 50 percent success rate of spine/disc surgery? Fortunately medical doctors are more and more likely to refer a disc patient to a chiropractor before the patient becomes a candidate for surgery and vise versa. Chiropractors know when an individual needs surgical intervention and will refer the patient to an M.D. when and if needed.

Chiropractors are taught to play detective until they get to the *root* of the problem, then treat the problem or refer the patient to another type of doctor. Chiropractors also treat a host of other problems besides back pain, including but not limited to headaches, sports injuries, carpal tunnel syndrome, fibromyalgia, and endocrine problems, and, like myself, chiropractors are proficient in nutritional matters.

It is wise to add a chiropractor to your entourage, your list of doctors whom you trust and see regularly. You may have a few medical doctors, including one who specializes in internal medicine, a gynecologist if you are a woman, a dermatologist, or maybe an ear-nose-throat doctor. Well, don't forget to check in with a chiropractor every so often. Chances are that you will need him or her at some point. So go out and find yourself a chiropractor.

Caloric Restriction

Caloric restriction may sound as if I am referring to dieting or losing weight. Nope. Recent studies have shown that staying on a low-calorie diet consistently and, well, forever, increases longevity. This is quite an amazing finding. There are more obvious benefits of caloric restriction, however, including lower rates of obesity and diabetes, but this new finding is much bigger than just losing weight for health benefits. The results of clinical studies show that specific metabolic mechanisms are at work when you limit your caloric intake to a certain number per day, on a continual basis, as a way of life. There is a supplement that is thought to mimic the actions on a cellular level (and with no weight loss) of caloric restriction. I will discuss that supplement later.

The people who live the longest lives (many of them in Okinawa, Japan) maintain a low but healthy weight. The average person in Okinawa takes in about 1,200 to 1,400 calories per day. They also have a very healthy diet that consists mainly of sweet potatoes, berries, and fish. I am not suggesting that everyone reading this book should reduce his or her daily intake of calories to this low level. First of all, everyone's metabolism is different, and we all have different caloric needs.

You must consider the amount of calories on average that you burn in a day. For example if you are a runner, you will need more calories than a sedentary person. Second, I just want you to become aware of the findings in current nutritional research. Again this fact is just amazing; that's all. The practice of caloric restriction is not a weight-loss system. It is a phenomenon that involves complicated happenings in the body on a cellular level that have to do with DNA, and I am not going to get into *that*.

All you need to know is that this is pretty much the first scientific discovery that has to do with life extension outside the subject of illnesses. Am I making sense? Okay, let's discuss how to take in fewer calories. It's simple. Just eat healthy. Cut out the crap. While you are at it, exercise, as I have already discussed. This way you will burn off some of those calories. Try to maintain a body weight that is healthy and not unhealthily low. Again I don't want anyone reading this to think I am suggesting a lifetime of dieting. I tell everyone to cut out the junk, never let yourself be hungry, and use common sense when choosing what you eat. That's it.

The latest research has given us yet another reason not to be overweight. Isn't extending your life worth it? Embrace this new fact, and look forward to your forthcoming efforts in promoting longevity and anti-aging.

CHAPTER 2

NUTRITIONAL SUPPLEMENTS

In this chapter I have only included some very powerful, as well as very important, supplements, ones that researchers will continue to study because of their surprising or successful results from recent studies. Most of you probably have never heard of at least one of these supplements. Hundreds of vitamins, minerals, and herbal supplements are available today. I discuss just a few that I consider powerful and worth taking, just to get you going and let you know what's out there.

This chapter, well, the entire book actually, is for informational purposes only. After reading it, get help from your own naturopathic or chiropractic doctor, one who specializes in nutrition, in conjunction with your medical doctor. This is very important because your M.D. must know which supplements you are taking and also give you the okay to take certain supplements if you take medications. You can then have a custom-made nutritional plan that is right for you.

Resveratrol and Curcumin

Resveratrol and curcumin are incredible anti-aging, cancer-fighting, and immune-supporting nutritional supplements you can find in most health food stores and even some grocery stores. A considerable amount of research has been done on these two beneficial supplements.

The first, resveratrol, is a compound extracted from grapes and the same compound found in wine. Recent studies show that resveratrol, when taken in supplement form, has the ability to encourage the lengthening of telomeres found in your DNA. I want to keep this book simple, so I don't want to get into the whole "DNA thing," but I will say that the longer the telomeres, the better. The length of your telomeres is directly linked to your predisposition to aging—in other words, the length of your life. Scientists are very excited about resveratrol and are working on many clinical trials that involve this supplement as well as its role in DNA and its exponential anti-aging potential.

Resveratrol is also a strong antioxidant and inflammation fighter. One last exciting piece of information about resveratrol is that studies show this supplement mimics the longevity effect of caloric restriction. Again I am not talking about a weight-loss effect, just the amazing effect of living longer. Now here is an important note on resveratrol. Although this compound comes from wine, drinking five or even twenty bottles per day won't work. Phew. I would hate to think that people are trying to drink their way to youth. It is virtually impossible to ingest the optimal amount of either grape juice or wine to reap the benefits of the nutritional compounds found in resveratrol.

The second nutritional supplement, curcumin, is an ancient spice found in Indian food. As with resveratrol, research has proven curcumin to be another strong cancer fighter as well as an excellent immune system booster. *The International Journal of Vitamin Nutritional Research* (1991, 61:364–69) states that curcumin also helps greatly in lowering one's cholesterol level and, more important, lowers bad (LDL) cholesterol while elevating good (HDL) cholesterol. Curcumin does this by interrupting the absorption of cholesterol, assisting the process of turning cholesterol into bile, and finally accelerating the elimination of bile. Exciting, right?

I know some of you are going to love this one. More than a few studies have shown that resveratrol and curcumin, when taken together in sort of a nutritional "cocktail," incredibly aid in the growth of hair and slow down hair loss. Ever see an Indian woman without gorgeous, long, thick, black hair? I doubt it. Is it just those great Indian genes, or could curcumin also have something to do with it?

I don't know about curcumin alone, and I already have covered the fact that no matter how much grape juice or wine you drink, you will not benefit from the longevity effects of resveratrol, but what about just eating a lot of grapes or drinking grape juice and taking curcumin? Is that enough to reap the benefit of hair growth? I am not completely sure yet. I probably will be able to tell you in my next book. Maybe I will travel to India before then. Regardless, studies show that when resveratrol and curcumin are combined and taken in supplement form, the effects on hair growth are great over time.

Now there is not much we can do yet about the graying of hair, ladies. Until some kind of nutritional discovery is made, we will have to resort to coloring, or just stick with a beautiful, silvery head of hair— which is just as beautiful as it is on all of you men out there.

Astaxanthin

Since I am going to give you more information on another nutritional supplement that is a phenomenal antioxidant, I need to explain a little bit about (without boring you) the natural aging (rotting) process that happens on a cellular level at a constant rate in our bodies. It is called oxidation. Oxidation is part of the natural process of aging and also contributes to lowered immune systems and increases one's susceptibility to illnesses. You cannot, as of yet, stop oxidation completely, but with the right compounds, enzymes, and foods, you can do a great deal to slow down the process considerably.

Free radicals cause oxidation of your cells. Think of free radicals as some of the worst enemies inside your body. You cannot eliminate them once and for all. It is more like an ongoing process in which you must constantly fend off these guys who do so much internal damage—damage you can see externally. You can fight this battle with the ingestion and application of antioxidants. An antioxidant is an oxidant-fighting nutrient found in the supplement resveratrol and the green, leafy vegetable kale. It is also found in berries (specifically blueberries, which are also super anti-inflammatories) and many other foods that actively fight off and break down free radicals and help to protect our cells from premature aging and illnesses. You must be proactive in eating the right power foods and taking the right nutritional supplements in order to fight a better battle against these bad guys.

Astaxanthin is a nutritional supplement that you probably never have heard of. It's an extremely powerful antioxidant, and if you were to take only one supplement per day while eating right, I would recommend this one. This compound is found in salmon and is made from algae and other marine plants. Astaxanthin is even more powerful than one of the popular ingredients used in skincare products, beta-carotene, which is found in carrots. Astaxanthin is also an extraordinary anti-inflammatory. Inflammation, on a cellular level, is involved in almost every known disease. You can help prevent inflammation, before diseases start to manifest, if you really pay attention to which foods you choose to eat.

So eat a lot of salmon, which is great for you for reasons other than what I am discussing now. You should not eat salmon every day; I would not recommend eating it every other day either. Twice per week is fine, but to get the sufficient amount of astaxanthin each day, you must not rely on eating salmon or algae. Take it in supplement form every day and of course with your doctor's knowledge.

Herbs and Cancer Prevention

Here we have a slightly tricky subject, that of herbs aiding in the prevention—and even sometimes the treatment—of certain cancers. Unbeknownst to most, herbs are naturally and highly active compounds, so I must caution you while informing you of their promising, positive effects. So here we go. I am going to introduce just a few excellent herbs for the sole purpose of examples.

Some skeptics choose not to believe in alternative care, alternative treatment, or alternative anything. The truth is that some "alternative" forms of prevention and/or treatment are becoming anything but alternative today. Studies have shown that under the supervision of a knowledgeable and experienced doctor, such as a naturopath or a medical doctor who specializes in this particular area of science, cancer can be slowed down or prevented by using different "cocktails" of herbs. This isn't to say that traditional methods don't work. I am *not* anti-medicine. I just want you to know that there are extra measures you can take.

Most people today feel they are at a lower risk of getting cancer because of advances in biotechnology, when, in fact, cancer rates have actually risen. The treatments may have gotten better, but there are ways in which you can help yourself fend off cancer in the first place. One way is through what I have already discussed, practicing healthy lifestyle habits. Another is through nutrition and another through herbs. I don't consider herbs to be a nutritional element. I think of herbs as more of natural medicine, and this is exactly the way I want you to think about herbs because of their potency. They are nothing to take lightly.

The first herb I want to discuss is called Chinese skullcap. The very powerful flavonoid found in Chinese skullcap is called baicalein. Chinese skullcap must be used with caution, as it is dangerous to take it without supervision by your specialized doctor. Be forewarned; many herbs come with side effects and can produce severe adverse reactions when ingested with other herbs and/or medications. You know those terrible commercials, the ones in which some kind of drug is promoted, and they show a person meandering happily through a green meadow, in hopes of distracting you from the liability clauses they must show across the screen at the end, warning you of all the serious side effects? Well, some herbs are no different. They are just as powerful as drugs and also come with risks. It works both ways; after all, where do you think drugs come from? Plants! Chinese skullcap is one of those herbs; it can give someone *serious* side effects that are quite common. Why am I telling you about it then? Because you can mention this herb to your naturopathic doctor who works alongside your medical doctor and get the correct dosages if you are a candidate for taking herbs.

Back to baicalein, which is contained in Chinese skullcap. It looks very promising with regard to not just the prevention of cancer but, more excitingly, the spread of cancer. Baicalein works by inhibiting certain enzymes from doing their normal jobs. These jobs, when done, are good for someone with no cancer cells. Normally you want the enzymes that are supposed to be in your body to do what they are supposed to do. This is not necessarily true for a cancer patient. Scientists now know that a cancer cell needs to bind with certain substances in order to grow, replicate, and spread. If the enzyme whose job it is to make these substances is inhibited, the substance won't be made and the cancer cell will be out of luck and eventually die. Pretty powerful stuff, right?

The next herb I want to tell you about is astragalus. This herb comes from a plant found in China and has been used in Chinese medicine for centuries. Today researchers in the US are studying astragalus to discover its role in cancer prevention. Astragalus is thought to induce the production of a chemical in your body called interferon, which is what your immune system needs to fight off cancer cells. In simpler terms, this herb is a super immune booster. So, you see, baicalein works to *inhibit*, while astragalus works to *promote*. They both do completely different things and have completely different roles, but these two herbs together can be promising for a specialized doctor who can do wonders for his or her cancer patient by concocting the right cancer-fighting herbal cocktail.

Prostate Cancer Prevention

If you are a woman reading this book, you can pass this information along to the male loved ones in your life. If you are a man, listen up.

For a man to do the best he can to prevent prostate cancer (which is rather common in men), first he must, of course, get an annual prostate exam, along with a blood test, after the age of forty, that looks for elevated levels of the prostate cancer marker PSA. He can, however, help prevent this form of cancer much earlier in life by eating lots of cruciferous veggies. Cruciferous vegetables include, but aren't limited to; broccoli, cauliflower, and watercress.

Another fruit/vegetable (it's actually a fruit, but I don't want to argue about it) a man needs to eat is the tomato. Eating a tomato a day is really not enough, though. Tomatoes contain a much needed compound called lycopene. To ingest enough lycopene to really be effective, and just as with some other nutrients I have mentioned, a man needs to ingest a lot of tomato sauce or tomato juice. I consider vegetable juice that contains tomatoes a real bang-for-your-buck food. It lacks fiber, but for people who find it difficult to take in all of their daily requirements of veggies (which is rising with further research), low-sodium V8 juice is perfect. You can take lycopene in supplement form every day, and it's readily available in grocery and health food stores.

Lastly, drinking pomegranate juice is crucial in the fight against prostate cancer—and aging, as it is an excellent anti-oxidant. Since drinking the juice of pomegranates means you're ingesting a higher amount of pomegranates, drink the juice. Drinking pomegranate juice from concentrate is fine. Try to buy a pure one, with less sugar and fewer calories. Avoid any juice that lists high fructose corn syrup in the first three ingredients. Pomegranate juice is expensive, so try to budget it in as a regular food staple. A great way to drink your V8 juice and have your pomegranates too is to pour equal amounts of V8 and pomegranate juice over ice in a large pitcher. In the summer throw a little lemonade in there too with a splash of Diet 7UP, and you'll have a refreshing, super-healthy, fun drink for you and your kids.

One last important fact is that men should avoid any amount of vitamin E that is over and above what is contained in a regular multivitamin. This is very important, updated news—well, updated to the general public. It's sad, but sometimes it takes forever for vital information to reach the "news." Taken in a higher-than-normal multivitamin dose, vitamin E accelerates precancerous cells of the prostate. So far research has found this to be true only for cancer of the prostate and not other cancers. I, myself, even being a woman, do not take any vitamin E other than what is in my daily multivitamin. I am just being cautious with it, since you never know what further research will turn up regarding other cancers. With that said, if you're a woman, you can break open a small vitamin E capsule and spread it around on your face before you go to bed at night. It might feel a little messy, but it's great for your skin when used topically.

Vitamin D3

Make sure to get your daily dose of vitamin D3. You will read about the importance of daily sunblock in the last chapter of this book. It seems ironic, but you must, every day, block out the sun's damaging rays, the same sun that supplies you with your daily dose of vitamin D3. The form of vitamin D that is so vital to your body is D3, not just D. There is a huge difference, which I won't get into now. I will just tell you that you get enough vitamin D through your regular diet and also your daily multivitamin, which you should take. Your body absorbs vitamin D3 from the sun. This vitamin is so important to your health that when you get your annual blood test, your doctor automatically (if he or she follows current guidelines) tests for vitamin D3 levels. Vitamin D3, absorbed through sunlight, assists your body in fighting off cancer and many other diseases. A lack of vitamin D3 is linked not only to cancer but also to bone diseases, heart disease, diabetes, and, as the latest research shows, Alzheimer's disease.

The FDA has even reevaluated vitamin D3. The, government-regulated FDA recently upped the recommended daily allowance to four hundred IUs per day. This amount, however, is hardly enough. Adults should take between two thousand and four thousand IUs per day. To get the necessary amount of D3 from sunlight alone, if you did not take D3 supplements, you would have to receive full-body exposure to the sun for fifteen minutes per day every day. That might sound pretty easy to do—just fifteen minutes per day—but unless you live in sunny southern California or Florida and you're able to slip your swimsuit on every day, you will not be able to get the adequate amount.

Children need eight hundred to one thousand IUs of vitamin D3 per day. Here's a tidbit for you. For the last twenty years, hospitals in Finland have given newborns four thousand IUs of vitamin D3 per day. They are twenty years ahead of us. I am not recommending that give your newborn anything. I was just blown away upon learning that Finland seems to be far more advanced in the research of vitamin D3 than the US. Again, getting advice from your, or your child's, medical doctor is advised before you take, or give to your child, any nutritional supplement.

So what about sunblock? As I said, you will get a good dose of that topic in a later chapter, but let's get back to sunny California and Florida. If you are lucky enough to live in either of these two warm states, or anywhere else that is considered sunny, and you do put your swimsuit on every day, and you are basically a full-fledged sun-worshiper, you are putting yourself at a high risk of skin cancer, also known as melanoma. Skin cancer is the most common cause of death among people age twenty-nine to forty-five, although if you're older than forty-five, you are not exactly out of the woods. There are still plenty of cases of skin cancer in older individuals. I know what you are thinking, and after you read Chapter 4, you will really be saying, "What the . . . ? Damned if you do, damned if you don't."

It really is quite simple. Wear your daily sunblock. Wear at least SPF 30 all over and every day. Take your daily vitamin D3, and you're good to go.

Vitamin C

As far as anti-aging goes, vitamin C is extremely beneficial when taken as a daily nutritional supplement. It also is used as a topical agent in high-quality facial creams and body lotions. When used topically and regularly, vitamin C helps speed up your skin's cell turnover rate and builds collagen. It also evens out skin tone while diminishing brown age spots.

Most of you probably already know about the incredible benefits vitamin C has on the immune system. I am sure your mother made you drink orange juice at the first sign of a cold or in the first stages of influenza. As it turns out, she was right. Scientific studies have proven that five hundred milligrams taken per hour (for an adult) at the onset of a cold or flu shortens the duration and/or the intensity of the illness. I find it interesting that we need to do scientific studies only to prove what people two hundred years ago already knew.

Let's talk about vitamin C and its contribution to longevity. Because of recent research (I know, research, research, research . . .), scientists are now discovering vitamin C's role in cancer prevention. What a bonus! So, yes, drink your orange juice just like your mother always told you and like her mother told her. Better yet, eat an orange every day, and if you're thirsty in the morning, stick to water. Oranges have a very high glycemic index, which means they are naturally high in sugar content, which spikes your blood sugar.

Now that I have mentioned water, stay away from those bottled vitamin waters that are flying off store shelves. These drinks are trendy and *seem* healthy. Vitamin waters, however, are very deceptive. Many, if not most, of these waters contain high fructose corn syrup, sometimes as their first or second ingredient. This means they contain extremely high amounts of sugar, which is not good for your teeth, waistline, or health in general. Another point is that the amount of vitamin C or any other vitamin in these drinks is minute. According to a 2002 *Tufts University Health & Nutrition Letter* article titled "Now, Bottled Water With Vitamins and Herbs," one popular brand of bottled vitamin water in particular was found, per serving, to contain an amount of vitamin C equivalent to that of two strawberries. So it's better to stick to good, old-fashioned plain water and not rely on vitamin water to reach your daily vitamin and mineral quota.

Selenium

As with astaxanthin, one of the most important nutritional supplements you should take is selenium. This strong antioxidant offers an abundance of health benefits, which makes it a valuable addition to your vitamin cabinet. Hm . . . a *vitamin* cabinet? I don't know about you, but I have one, and you should have one too. You probably have a medicine cabinet, and that's where you might throw in a few bottles of vitamins, right? Well, hopefully after reading this book you will have at least separated your vitamins from your medicines by having two different cabinets. The one you keep your medications in will shrink while your new vitamin cabinet grows.

My closest friends know my medicine cabinet is very small. In it I keep one bottle of Advil, one bottle of children's Motrin (I have a nine-year-old), children's Mucinex, a bottle of Pedialyte, a box of *Star Wars* Band-Aids, Bactine spray, and bug-bite anti-itch lotion. That's it. Now ask me what's in my vitamin cabinet, and I will not even attempt to list everything in there for fear of boring you. Someone like me must have a designated place just for nutritional supplements, and I am hoping you soon will have one too. Maybe over time there will be less of a need for you to take so many medications.

Why is selenium so great? For starters, in terms of anti-aging, selenium is a super free-radical fighter and a cancer fighter. Selenium actually inhibits the growth of cancer tumors, and if you take two hundred micrograms per day, your chances, over time, of dying from cancer decrease by 30 to 40 percent. Another area this supplement has a role in is diabetes. Selenium helps diabetics by indirectly stimulating the uptake of glucose (sugar), thereby acting like insulin. Selenium is a regulator. To keep this simple, I will just say that selenium regulates very important pathways that are associated with the regulation of blood sugar. This is vital to diabetics and hypoglycemic patients.

One last fact about selenium is that studies have revealed a correlation between dementia patients and low blood levels of—you guessed it—selenium. I don't know about you, but this last bit of information would be enough for me to run out and ask my doctor for the okay and start taking selenium today. I obviously already did that, though, so now it is your turn. Set up your vitamin cabinet today, and make sure this supplement ends up in there.

Krill Oil and Joint Health

Being a chiropractor, I have a great deal of interest in joint health and arthritis. Arthritis affects a high percentage of the senior population, as well as athletes and people under sixty years of age. There is an abundance of drugs out there prescribed by medical doctors to help alleviate the pain and swelling, but the effects are usually temporary, and sometimes these drugs don't work—all of these toxic drugs for nothing.

Maybe you have heard of the supplement glucosamine chondroitin sulfate, which improves joint function over time when taken consistently. Another supplement that has similar effect is krill oil. Krill oil comes from krill, which are tiny crawdad-like creatures that live near the bottom of the ocean (although I see huge groups of them floating on the surface of the ocean each time my son and I go whale-watching; the whales eat them). Krill oil is a major omega-3 provider and, when taken every day in the form of a three-hundred-milligram supplement, can greatly reduce joint inflammation. Joint inflammation could be— and in fact probably is—your main source of pain if you suffer from arthritis. Just a quick lesson—any illness or disease ending in "–itis" means "inflammation of . . . " If you suffer from arthritis, you suffer from inflammation along with degeneration of your joints.

Make sure not to confuse krill oil with fish oil. Krill oil is different, even though krill are considered a type of fish. Confused yet? Well, you can take fish oil too. I recommend one thousand to two thousand milligrams per day for cardiovascular benefits; fish oil also helps to lower bad (LDL) cholesterol. You need three hundred milligrams per day, and no more, of krill oil to receive the joint health benefits of anti-inflammation. If you are not sure which supplement you should trust for your joints, ask your doctor whether you should give krill oil a try. As I have said before, he or she should always know which herbs, vitamins, and supplements you are taking.

CHAPTER 3

FOODS

"You are what you eat," or so the saying goes. Well, you definitely are a product of what you eat. Let's go with that.

As in the last chapter, which covers some of my favorite nutritional supplements, I could not, and would not, list in this book all of the wonderfully healthy foods to eat in the world. That is just not necessary to bring across the points I need to bring to you while passing on important information you need to know regarding food, anti-aging, and longevity. In this book I include the real bang-for-your-buck foods that are loaded with antioxidants, and/or may be disease-specific-busting foods. I have picked the favorites of anti-aging researchers and scientists who are witnessing firsthand what these awesome foods can do and what the bad ones can do too. These bad "foods" deserve even much more criticism than they have previously received.

If you are already following what you consider a healthy diet, use this chapter as a supplemental guide (I like that word, "supplement"). If you are eating crap, use this chapter as a motivational startup guide. After reading this book, I want you to clean out your fridge. Go to your favorite grocery store and stay far away—I repeat, *stay away*—from the middle aisles, which are stocked with pure junk, and come back with fresh and/or frozen (frozen is just as nutritious, really) fruits and veggies—lots and lots of veggies—and reload your fridge.

Add to your daily diet the tasty age-fighters that you will read about in this chapter, and remove the unwanted ones from your pantry and your mouth forever.

Sugar

Sugar, unfortunately, is an enormous contributor to the process of human deterioration—more specifically, premature aging. Sugar is, by far, the hardest part of the battle for me. I love sugar. I love it in every form that exists—cupcakes, candy, white bread, white rice, whatever, as long as it involves sugar. If this sounds like you, then you will not like what you are about to hear, if you haven't heard it already.

We all know that sugar is not good for us. While growing up, we had it drilled into us that sugar rots our teeth, makes us fat, makes children hyper, and in large quantities will give us type 2 diabetes. Sugar has gotten a bad rap, but researchers are finding that it is even worse for us than previously thought.

Here is how sugar works its evil onto us. When you ingest sugar, it breaks down into molecules that attach themselves to protein fibers in your bloodstream. This process is called glycation, and as far as aging goes, this action is the culprit in the breakdown of collagen fibers in your skin. More glycation means more inflammation, which leads to more oxidation and ultimately more aging. Glycation is also a process involved in the development of type 2 diabetes and cardiovascular disease.

So please, at the very least, cut down your sugar intake or eliminate sugar from your diet entirely, which is not easy. To eliminate sugar entirely, you must shy from anything made with white, refined flour, and all forms of alcohol. White flour, like alcohol, basically turns into sugar in your body, and that's not pretty. If you eat a lot of white rice and white breads and also like to drink a glass of wine each night, you will have to make a few sacrifices (as if sacrificing chocolate, cupcakes, and jelly beans weren't enough!). Besides cutting out the crap from your diet, you also must switch from white rice to brown rice and your white bread to 100 percent whole grain bread. The label on any whole grain item must state "100 percent whole grain," or it is not whole grain at all. Whole grains are a very important part of a healthy diet. So start switching. Add popcorn to your diet as a snack, for when you get the nighttime munchies while watching *Once Upon a Time* or *Modern Family*. Popcorn is a whole grain and helps you meet your daily fiber quota. If you buy the packaged kind that pops in the microwave, buy a brand that contains no trans fats and states "light" on the label.

Well, there you have it. Premature aging is just one more reason to kick the sugar habit for good.

Butter and Oils

There certainly are many different "butters" out there, including one type of real butter that I like, but first I'd like to admit that I, myself, am sometimes guilty of consuming substitutes that are not really natural or healthy. For example I buy diet, caffeine-free soda, one that does not exactly taste like Diet Coke or Pepsi because it is an off-brand and has Splenda in it. I am okay with consuming a limited amount of Splenda, while I am *not* okay with the old-time artificial sweeteners aspartame and saccharine, which are chemicals. Splenda, being chemically treated or altered, is made from sugar, and for now is considered safe for children. Still I try to limit all artificial sweeteners from my family's diet. Wow, maybe I should have put all of this in my previous section on sugar. Let's get back to butter and oils.

The point I want to make now is that all of those "butter" spreads in the grocery stores—which taste anything like butter and are supposed to be better for you—aren't. They are not better butter (sorry for the tongue twister). As their second ingredient, these spreads usually contain partially hydrogenated fats or oils, which are the worst. If you must choose a spread, make sure it is *not* margarine. Margarine became popular back in the '80s, before all of these other spreads came out, and is filled with trans fats, which are very toxic on a cellular level. Real butter, of course, is not good for you either because it contains pure saturated fat, the kind that re-solidifies in your arteries, clogging them like nothing else can. What I put on my toast in the morning is 100 percent real, whipped butter. If you eat whipped butter, teaspoon for teaspoon you actually use less butter than if you use regular non-whipped butter, and that is why the calorie and fat gram counts on the container are lower. That's the only difference—it is whipped. Try to remember to leave the butter out for fifteen minutes to soften it. Whipped cream cheese is healthier and lower in calories than low-fat cream cheese for the same reasons, and fat-free cream cheese tastes so bad that I would rather eat a plain bagel.

Regarding oils, it is rather simple. All you need to know and remember when choosing cooking or salad oil is to buy either canola or olive oil. These two oils are good for you. I keep both in my kitchen because some dishes—for example, hash browns—don't taste quite right when cooked with olive oil. Ditto for baking cookies and cakes. When I need a cooking spray, I buy a generic brand with canola oil being the only ingredient. There are a few other oils that are okay, but it really does start to get a little confusing, so just focus on the two oils discussed here, and your kitchen, taste buds, and heart will love you.

Coffee—Thumbs Up

Listen up everyone, *drink coffee*. I repeat (unless your own doctor advises against it), *drink your coffee*. You should be reaping the antioxidative rewards of coffee by drinking *at least* a few big mugs of it per day. Oxidation, caused by free radicals, is an unfortunate and deteriorating process that occurs inside your body. Having your cup of Joe every day is just one way by which you can slow down this ugly process, and it's a great one. This should be easy because drinking coffee every morning is something most of you already do. In fact, Americans get more antioxidants from coffee than anything else. Unfortunately most of you don't know it, and I am informing you now. You need even more than your daily cup. So just increase your daily quota (a word I like and use often). Have an extra cup in the morning then meet up with your friends at Starbucks after the evening rush hour instead of going to happy hour at your nearest bar.

Here is a bit of info I'll bet you didn't know. Your liver loves coffee. Coffee (for this entire section I am including decaf, which is just as healthy and effective) helps the liver do its job, which is to filter out any and all toxins from the body as best it can. Coffee supports this very important function.

Research shows that people who drink a good amount of coffee daily have a lower chance of getting type 2 diabetes because of coffee's ability to regulate blood sugar. Here's something else. It may be because of the caffeine in regular coffee, but coffee also has a positive effect on those suffering from depression. This last piece of info is for any students out there reading this. I know from past experience and from studies I've read that drinking regular (not decaf) coffee while studying helps to retain the information needed for the next day's exam. Oh, and by the way, I aced all of my exams in college.

So there you go. You no longer need to feel guilty about drinking too much coffee.

Alcohol—Thumbs Down

I want to set everyone straight regarding alcohol. Over the last few years there has been chatter out there concerning whether alcohol is good for you. Come on. Good for you? Give me a break. There are much better ways to "relax" your heart. A glass of wine or a beer once in a while is fine, but the talk about having one to two drinks per day being a good thing is just wrong. Forget alcohol. It is bad for you and especially bad for women.

For both men and women, alcohol is a major contributor to heart disease as well as disease of the liver (sorry, but coffee is not going to get you out of this one). What I am going to tell you now might not sound right, with all of the other conflicting advice out there regarding alcohol, but here it is (and this holds true for only women). If you consistently have more than three drinks per week of any type of alcohol, you are four times more likely to fight the ugly battle of breast cancer. So, no, it does not stop at the liver, and alcohol (even red wine) is not good for you, like many of you previously thought. Now you must think about your heart, your liver, *and* cancer when it comes to the decision regarding whether to drink on a regular basis.

It really does not seem fair that women have to worry about cancer because of drinking and men don't. Well, mark my words. It is only a matter of time before scientists find other cancers caused by or aggravated by alcohol—not that we women want men to suffer too. I am merely suggesting that your male loved ones also should beware of the fact that for something as toxic as rotted fruit, potatoes, rice, or whatever it was that was chosen to *rot* in order to make the alcohol, it should come as no surprise that alcohol causes major illnesses of many kinds over time.

Some of you may not know exactly what alcohol is, or how it is made. Did you know that thousands of years ago, and maybe even still today in certain parts of the world, people would look forward to eating disgustingly rotted fruit that had been picked off the ground in the hopes of getting high? They were getting drunk. Rotten foods are toxic. You can get a reaction from eating rotten fruit, the same reaction in fact as when you drink a glass of any kind of alcohol. You get this drunken reaction because you get poisoned by the chemicals that developed during the natural rotting process. Even though your drink of choice, whether it's a Cosmopolitan or a Merlot, is rotted in factories or beautiful, romantic wineries and then bottled and wrapped with a nice label and given a name, it still is what it is, spoiled juices from rotted foods.

So, please *do* ignore the "Whew, I can drink away now. Studies show alcohol is good for me" myth.

Is Red Meat for Cavemen?

First, I have to tell everyone how much I enjoyed reading *Skinny Bitch* by Rory Freedman and Kim Barnouin. In fact, I think I'll read it again after I finish writing this book. Their book is in your face and to the point, very refreshing and informative. I loved it. You too must read *Skinny Bitch*. The book is not really about being skinny at all but makes the point that the benefit of being nicely skinny is what you will receive if you eat and live a certain way, which by the way does not involve "the ancient, caveman-like ways of eating the rotted carcasses of animals." The book also states that "those animals of thousands of years ago were not grossly mistreated and tortured before being slaughtered as they are in today's society here in the US."

After reading *Skinny Bitch*, I became highly motivated not to just stop eating red meat, but I became one of those people who refuse to eat anything that had parents. This was pretty easy for me, because I do not particularly enjoy sitting at the table with a filet of anything in front of me. I actually love good veggies, salads, and fruits. Since I was already well aware of the serious increased health risks associated with eating meat (especially red meat) on a regular basis, it did not take much for the book to convince me to give up meat altogether. I must admit, though, that I have since caved (no pun intended). I have, however, remained vigilant in my mini-revolution against the meat industry by preaching to my family and friends. They listen, some slightly reluctantly, to me rattle on about how they are indirectly supporting the inhumane treatment of animals through their purchases, of even eggs, from the grocery store. I now only buy local free-range eggs, and I am now seriously thinking about raising my own backyard chickens. Thank you, *Skinny Bitch*.

I am not suggesting that you refrain from eating all meat or even all red meat. My goal is to make you more aware of just how much protein your body really needs and that there are many forms of protein other than meat. Consuming red meat is now linked to a decrease in longevity, or, in other words, mortality. That's right. There are clinical, follow-up studies being done right now. Results are already coming in, and you will be hearing more about this in the coming months (as I write this I it is now March 2012).

I suggest that you cut *way* down on meat, especially red meat, because it is high in saturated fat and also because of the recent results of the studies being done today, as explained above. So how much protein do we really need? Well, some protein every day is certainly a good idea. When it comes down to how much protein should be on your dinner plate, I am going to tell you to follow the popular Mediterranean diet. This diet recommends consuming a small portion of protein in the form of meat that is no bigger than the size of your palm; for your child, the portion should be the size of his or her palm. This amount of protein once per day or at one meal per day is enough. Too much protein is hard on your kidneys, but most important, you are leaving less room for the truly important foods that you need to eat each day to achieve longevity.

To live longer while looking and feeling younger, you must concentrate on vegetables, legumes (beans), fruits, and whole grains. If you don't believe me, check out the new USDA Food Pyramid, which is now a Food Plate. It certainly is not the same one taught in schools when I was a kid, thank God. Shaped like a pie, it has changed entirely and shows that protein is the least important food group, with the biggest pieces of the pie being whole grains, then veggies, fruits, and legumes. Yeah! It's about time. My son is getting positive, nutritional reinforcement from school. It took long enough. So anyway, this is no longer opinion; it is considered fact, accepted by the public. You need a lot less protein than previously thought.

When choosing which protein to feed your family, select lean meat, such as turkey, pork, chicken, lean beef, or the best protein, I feel, fish, especially salmon, which is high in omega-3. Here again I am going to mention the Mediterranean diet, of which I am an advocate. When I use the term "diet," I refer to an ongoing, regular, dietary routine. I am not talking about a diet meant to lose weight. The Mediterranean diet is the best regular, everyday, lifestyle diet out there to follow—if you choose to follow one, that is.

Egg Whites

Since we are on the subject of *protein*, I thought it best to bring up one "super food" that I hope to turn you on to, the simple egg white. Egg whites are super because of the protein they pack into their tiny shell. The white of the egg is a complete protein, meaning if you eat it you don't need to eat proteins from other sources to meet your daily protein quota. Some proteins are actually partial proteins. For example, legumes are considered a partial protein but are a complete protein if eaten with rice. I also like the fact that there is zero fat in an egg white and very few calories.

Egg whites are truly one of those bang-for-your-buck foods. Of course, the entire egg is good for you, and the fat in the yolk is considered a "good" fat, if not eaten every day, sort of like an avocado.

A three-egg omelet once per week for breakfast is fine and should be considered a treat. If you want the bang-for-your-buck benefit, eat only the white of the egg, and you can eat one, two, or three every day. I do. I boil a dozen at a time, keep them in my fridge, and eat the whites as snacks. Egg-white-only omelets are great too. Add to the whites a tiny amount of Canadian bacon (it's basically ham), a *sprinkle* of goat or feta cheese, chopped onion, bell pepper, or whatever. You can get very creative with eggs.

Greek Yogurt

Yes, I know, Greek yogurt has become trendy, but with good reason. It is a powerhouse of protein compared to other yogurts, with the added benefit of calcium. I am referring to *plain*, *nonfat* Greek yogurt. The ones with added crap like sugar and full fat are not worth talking about. There is no favorable protein-to-calorie/fat ratio in those. So stick with the plain, nonfat variety. I mix mine with about half a cup of high-fiber cereal such as All-Bran, along with berries. Sometimes I mix in flax seed or pineapple chunks. Other times I just eat it plain. The texture is also what makes Greek yogurt so good, so I don't mind it plain with nothing in it at all. Lucky me.

Pomegranate Seeds

There is a fairly new (by the time you read this it will no longer be considered new, and I am going as fast as I can with this book) snack product being sold right now in most chain grocery stores. It is an abso-lutely brilliant idea, pomegranate seeds in a container. The name of the product is POM POMs Fresh Arils pomegranate seeds. These seeds are packed airtight in a cute little container with a re-sealable lid, and a foldable plastic spoon is included. The container holds 4.3 ounces of seeds, which contain only one hundred calories. When I found them for the first time, I threw about fifty packages into my cart. The lady behind the counter must have thought I was crazy. When I got home, I put most of them in the freezer. Turns out they are even better frozen. They are very convenient to take with you to work, to the park, or wherever.

I wrote about pomegranates and pomegranate juice in a previous chapter to tell you about their fantastic cancer-fighting and free-radical-fighting capabilities, which also make these seeds a great anti-aging snack. This packaged snack is super because you also get fiber from the seeds. Have you ever sat down to eat a pomegranate? Remember when you were a kid and your mother would have to put down a towel first? It can be quite messy not to mention time consuming. I hope you give this snack a try.

Apples

"Apples? A part of my daily diet?" You bet. Our ancestors knew a thing or two when they told us, "An apple a day keeps the doctor away." Two apples per day is even better. The variety of apple does not matter, as long as it is round, came off a tree, and has a peel. In other words I am referring to all varieties of apples here. The cancer-fighting abilities of apples, along with the antioxidative polyphenol called quercetin found in the apple, makes the apple an important part of your daily diet. Don't forget that the peel holds fiber too, so don't peel your apples. Here is a tidbit for any calorie watchers reading this. Apples are a negative-calorie food. This simply means that by the time you have chewed up and digested your apple, you will have burned more calories than the apple contains. An average-size apple contains eighty calories and tastes so good. Who doesn't like apples?

If you worry about pesticides on your apples and don't want to pay for organic, don't peel them. Simply wash your apples with water or a with a fruit spray, which you can find in most supermarkets. You also can purchase fruit sprays online. They work, they are harmless, they don't leave any taste behind, and they are made chemical free, of course, using citrus compounds along with coconut or palm oil.

It is important to note that apple juice is not exactly good for you. One cup contains many apples, without the fiber for digestion but with a lot of calories from sugar. So eat your apples. Don't drink them.

I promise that you will be reading more about apples in the future, as many studies are being performed on apples and their anti-aging effects. So go out and get yourself and your family lots of apples today.

Walnuts

I hope you like walnuts. If you do, that's great. If you don't, try to find a way to enjoy eating them. You probably have heard that nuts are good for you. Well, walnuts are the best nuts to choose and are another one of my super foods. Here again, with the walnut, I picked a superb cancer fighter. According to the American Association for Cancer Research, along with the results of follow-up studies, a daily dose of walnuts in your diet helps ward off and slow down the growth of cancerous tumors with unique compounds called phytosterols.

An added bonus is that the walnut is the nut with the highest level of antioxidant properties. On a daily basis, you only need to eat a very small amount of walnuts, about two ounces. Don't overdo it. Walnuts are extremely high in fat calories. If you eat too many every day, you might end up, well, fat.

By now you might be thinking, *Gosh, every food in this book is about cancer and/or antioxidants.* Yes, that is why I picked these particular foods. There are many other foods that either help to prevent or slow down cancer, but as I said before, I need not list them all. This little book has in it some of the best and is just intended to get you going. Now go buy yourself some walnuts.

YOUR SKIN

I kept this chapter even shorter than the others, because whatever you decide to do with the previous chapters eventually will show in your skin. It's that simple. This book *is*, after all, titled *From the Inside Out* for a reason. Your skin is the biggest part of the "out." Other than ways to protect your skin from aging and cancer, I've included advice on a few things you can do to keep your skin feeling pampered and looking good in the process. I hope you try them, and I hope you like them. Most important, I want you to realize when reading this chapter that while using avocados on your face is optional, wearing sunblock isn't.

Sunblock

I woke up this morning to a beautiful, sunny day. After I finish writing this section on sunblock, I will happily and religiously practice my daily morning ritual, even in the winter, of slathering SPF 30 to 70 all over my face, neck, arms, hands, and any other parts of my body that may be exposed. I reapply sunblock on my hands three to four times per day at least. Soon, because of the coming summer season (remember, as I write this it is mid-March), the sunblock lotion will be covering my legs underneath self-tanning lotion. I keep sunblock in my car, and I carry a tube in my purse. It's pretty much with me everywhere I go. I am a sunblock fanatic, and you should be too.

You know all of those anti-aging and cancer claims, the ones that blame the sun on everything from wrinkles and brown spots to malignant moles? They are all true. As a child and adolescent growing up in Southern California, I worshiped the sun. Smothered in Hawaiian Tropic tanning oil, my sister, my friends, and I would "lay out," as they called it back then, on our flat patio roof and literally fry ourselves. As if that weren't good enough, we also would use those sun reflectors made from tin foil, or something like it, to soak in even more of the sun's rays. We couldn't get enough! Back in the '80s even grocery stores sold those things. No one ever tried to stop us. The most any of our parents said to us was, "If you start getting burned, put some SPF 4 sunscreen on." Then we would say, "No way. My burn will turn to a tan color in a day or two and look so good!"

Back then no one really knew about, or least talked about, the dangers of the sun's rays. Being tan, it seemed, was equated with being healthy. "Oh, your deep, dark tan looks so great. You have such a healthy glow" is what I would say to anyone with a great tan. I don't know exactly what hit me around the time I turned twenty, but I started to religiously use SPF 15 to 30 sunblock on my face and neck each day and stopped sunbathing all together. At the beach it was full-body sunblock, a hat, and an umbrella. My friends made fun of me then. They don't now. I am a proud forty-three-year-old with not one age spot and very few wrinkles, and I credit my using sunblock for that. Sure, I use anti-aging creams on my face and neck, but those only help to a certain degree. Because of the abuse I put my skin through while growing up, I have skin checks each year, and I am pretty confident that I am safe from malignant melanoma, which is the deadliest form of cancer among people age twenty-nine to forty-five.

There are many misconceptions regarding the sun's damaging rays related to cancer and/or aging. Most people don't realize that an accumulation of just ten to fifteen minutes a day of sun received by taking several short walks to and from the car, for example, is damaging. This kind of exposure to the sun is called incidental sun exposure. One year of incidental sun exposure is equivalent to an entire week of sunbathing in Hawaii sans sunblock. This might not sound like much to you, but as you get older and begin your quest to reverse any sun damage done to your skin over the years, any bit of damage becomes a lot.

Another misconception is that on cloudy days there is no need to wear sunblock. This belief couldn't be any more wrong. Just as many harmful, aging rays come through those clouds from the sun as they do on the clearest of days. Because of a cloud cover, you might feel a false sense of security, thinking you could not possibly be getting any sun, when in fact, the rays are bouncing and reflecting off the moisture in the clouds and exposing you even more. Everyone I know, including myself, has at some point in his or her life (probably as a teen) received a bubbling, blistering sunburn on the beach on one of those cloudy summer days.

So if you really desire healthy, cancer-free, wrinkle-free, younger-looking skin, you must be diligent with your use of sunblock. Don't forget to teach your children that they too can still have fun all summer long in the sun while wearing sunblock.

Anti-Aging Topical Skincare

Did you know that your skin is your largest organ? Not only is it an organ, and the largest, but also it's the one that goes exposed and unprotected and is vulnerable. I just discussed the importance of protection with sunblock, so now let's discuss *reversing* sun damage with a little help from your local drugstore or my personal favorite cosmetic and skincare chain, Sephora.

You see the ads for new, high-tech, anti-aging facial creams every time you flip through a fashion magazine. There are so many of these products on the market that it is difficult to pick one. I must tell you from experience that they do work. I have used, and still use, many of them. These creams all pretty much work the same way. They contain special ingredients (which I am not going to list here) that fade brown spots, even out skin tone, smooth wrinkles, and firm the skin. Don't go crazy trying to figure out which one to pick. Just pick one, actually two, because you also are going to use a daytime facial cream that contains—you guessed right—sunblock. Many daytime facial creams contain SPF 30, which I recommend. You also will use a night-time cream that claims to make you look younger. It will; trust me. You don't have to go to Sephora and spend eighty dollars a pop for one of these wonderful creams. You can find plenty of anti-age creams at your local grocery store or pharmacy that work just as well. There are a few wrinkle-erasing skincare lines in particular that I love. For starters, Olay, which used to be thought of as "Grandma's face cream," has become very advanced while retaining its signature moisturizing capabilities. The other line I recommend is RoC, which contains retinol and helps re-texturize the skin. Two other good ones are Revlon and L'Oreal.

Many great products are available for your body too. After all, you don't want to have lizard-like, aged skin on your body while sporting a youthful-looking, cared-for face and neck. When I get out of the shower, I like to use a body lotion that contains exfoliating alpha-hydroxy acids, which also make it very moisturizing. I use AmLactin-5, which contains lactic acid and is sold in drugstores. This lotion is for dry skin, which mine is. It has a rather strong, chemical-like scent upon application, but the odor disappears rather quickly and is worth the smell anyway. I then slather on my sunblock of course. At night a heavy cream that includes white petroleum jelly as its main ingredient, such as Gold Bond Healing Cream, does wonders on hands, feet and elbows.

When you go out into the sun for extended periods of time, on vacations for example, always wear sunglasses for extra protection. A hat would be great too. Cover up! There is a good reason why women two hundred years ago had great skin, even before SPF lotions were invented. Ever hear of a parasol? Actually, women in previous generations always wore hats too, along with white gloves on even the hottest of days. I'm guessing these women, even back then, knew a thing or two about the damaging effects of the sun.

Avocados on My Face? Really?

Yes, really. I am choosing to let you in on one of my little secrets. I have discovered that using avocados on your skin transforms its texture and smoothes it out while giving it an incredible amount of moisture. I am referring to your face here. It really is not feasible— and would be very messy—to bathe in avocados.

Avocados are a good exfoliant due to the enzymes they contain. They also break down oil while depositing enzymes deep into the pores, which helps strengthen the interlocking fibers that make up collagen. The huge amount of fat in avocados is a bonus that delivers moisture and feels like heaven on your skin. Wow. No high-tech, advanced formulas here. This mask is just pure, fresh, mashed-up avocado slathered all over your face and neck. Rest for fifteen minutes or so, rinse off, and you're done. Trust me, after a few months of twice-per-week treatments, you will see and feel a difference in the softness of your face.

If you feel tempted to eat your avocado, envision the number six hundred in your mind, because that is how many fat calories are in one large avocado. Stick to just a slice of this "good" fat as a salad topper. Better on your face than your waistline, right?

CHAPTER 5

THE PSYCH-HEALTH CONNECTION

How do you like this book so far? It's quick, easy reading, right? Are you feeling motivated to take charge of your chronological/biological clock? I love this chapter, as it completes the big picture, and that is why I left it for last. After reading it you should be able to answer the questions "Am I *really* healthy? Have I been doing everything necessary to ensure myself a long and healthy life?"

Whether or not you have doesn't matter. What matters now is that you have in front of you, all contained into this short book, the ways in which you can change your routine into a healthier one. Reading this last chapter is so important, because it covers not just how to improve your mental health but also your overall health. What your mind thinks and does your body follows, even on a subconscious, microscopic, cellular level. So read this chapter in its entirety, even the part about falling in love, and take it to heart—literally.

Keeping the Mind Young

For some time the general public has known that the more you read and learn, the better chance your mind has of staying memory-loss-free as you enter your golden years. Not only is this true, but surprisingly researchers are finding out that this need for mindful exercise starts at a much earlier age than previously thought.

Scientists are discovering that a lot starts to happen to one's brain around the age of forty. Ah, no wonder I've been losing my car keys; I just turned forty-three. From the age of forty through sixty, your brain starts to slowly but surely lose its ability to retain and recall information. In other words you start to lose your memory. During this time period, you need to keep the circuitry in your brain active. You must open up new synapses in your brain by regularly engaging in thinking activities. Any activities that require you to think, learn, or study are great. These sorts of activities can include everything from puzzles and chess, to Internet poker and blanket bingo. The important common denominator in these games is that they keep the mind challenged. Keep your mind stimulated, and you should suffer less memory loss as you reach old age. Old age can be and should be fun!

Hold on now. Forty, fifty, and even sixty are not considered old age, you might be thinking. Well, don't get angry with me, but it is all relative, right? I am just being realistic. Hey, I am forty-three. My age is my age. I am not old, but I am no spring chicken either. I am completely comfortable with accepting my age, and you should be comfortable accepting yours too.

With all of that said and read, all of you out there who are seeking a second career through a new degree or vocational training will accomplish more than just a fatter, future bank account. You are paving your way to a happier, healthier, and younger mind. Hopefully, through even further research, we can, on a mental level, make sixty the new forty.

Sunshine

This subject hits home with me. I ask myself every day, *What the heck was I thinking?* I am referring to my decision to move my family across the US, three thousand miles away from beautiful, sun-smothered Southern California, to settle into a rather dark and dismal part of the northeast—namely Connecticut. I was thinking about the seasons at the time. As a child, I never knew what true seasons were like. Okay, Connecticut *is* beautiful in the fall, with its leaves and all. During the rest of the year, however, its beauty takes on more of a greenish-brown hue, involving lots of mud, except when there is snow—lots of snow. Give yourself enough time here, and you too will find yourself wanting to take a paintbrush to every living green and brown (did I mention brown?) thing in your yard in a desperate attempt to turn it into Disneyland. Oh, and you'll want to paint the sky blue too. If you grew up in a sunny state like California, you tend to think that blue is the color the sky is supposed to be. There is one more thing lacking here in Connecticut. The sun! On an actual nice, sunny day here, you are expected to take advantage of today's sunshine, because it probably will not be there tomorrow.

Some people here don't seem to mind all of Connecticut's dreary, cloudy days. Things got a little better for me while watching, with much enthusiasm, my new sunroom being built. The only problem is that my sunroom isn't very sunny without the sun. Go figure.

Two hundred years ago, in a time when medicine was limited, an ill person was subjected to a form of "medicine" then called "supportive therapy." This was a regular practice, not only for mental hospitals but also for the healing of any and all physical illnesses. Supportive therapy meant simply putting an ill patient into the warm sunshine for several hours per day. Doctors back then were on to something.

There is a mental disorder, more common than you might think, called seasonal effective disorder. This illness can be severe but is temporary and mainly affects people who live in darker, colder climates such as Washington and Alaska—especially Alaska, where the winters are very long and the days are almost nonexistent during certain times of the year when the darkness takes over. The people who succumb to this disorder are extremely sensitive to the effect that limited sunlight has on nearly everyone. These sufferers become not just depressed but clinically depressed to the point where they may need to take medication.

As far as supportive therapy goes, even if there were no direct, obvious effects on those ill patients' physical symptoms, through the sunlight's positive effects on mental and emotional wellbeing, at least some of those patients would have felt better and become happier, thereby allowing the mind-body connection to work and facilitating those patients' abilities to actually get better physically.

The mind, you see, is a very powerful entity all its own. It is so powerful, in fact, that scientists are working nonstop at trying to figure out how we can stop invading viruses or mutating cancerous cells in their tracks just by thinking about it. Visual imagery is a field of science and medicine that is very real. My own father beat his debilitating facial pain caused by trigeminal neuralgia through sheer visual imagery. He uses no drugs. This is huge. I know I am getting off track here, so back to sunshine.

Sunshine has a direct, calming, uplifting, and literally warming effect on your psychological wellbeing while having an indirect effect on you physically. The next time you feel down in the dumps, get to your favorite sunlit spot quickly, and please wear sunblock.

Stress and Hair Loss

Hair loss is a topic that is a sore spot for most men, although women experience hair thinning too. We all have seen men, sometimes as young as the age of thirty, starting to go bald. As we age, losing hair is a natural, normal process that for the most part is genetic. Your DNA handed down from Mom and Dad decide when and how much hair you will lose. Just because it is natural, however, does not mean you have to like it or put up with it.

There are products out there for men, such as Rogaine, that might work, and there is a version available for women too. You can always try a hair transplant. I have seen the before and after, and not in pictures. Trust me. Hair transplants do not work. The before was definitely better. One man I know of suffered horrible, visible scabs on his scalp just to have any little hairs that were transplanted fall out months later. For women there are many different brands of hair extensions that are glued or sewn near the scalp. Well, I have seen these too, not the before but the after. Again they're not a great idea. What I thought was an envious head of thick, shiny hair longer than my own (which took five years to grow) on one of my new friends was actually a head of thick, long, beautiful hair extensions. Yes, they looked great, but while meeting her for the first time at a luncheon with mutual friends, I noticed she had to keep excusing herself so she could scratch her head in the ladies room. I later learned from her that these extensions are just not worth it. Her scalp was in a constant state of disease. Yes, the pulling, the scratching, and the buildup of dead skin cells on the scalp left there because of her inability to brush through the extentions where the hair meets the scalp led to infected lesions (the same kind that hair transplants leave on men). Sounds nice and clean, right?

Better to focus on ways of fighting off hair loss, I hope you are thinking.

With that, I will now tell you how to help prevent accelerated hair loss. You cannot prevent hair loss completely, but you can slow it down considerably if you get serious about health. As you might recall (unless you are over forty, ha ha), earlier in this book I talked briefly about the two supplements that studies showed to be promising in preventing or slowing down hair loss. These supplements, both resveratrol and cur-

cumin, I take each day, along with twenty-two other nutritional supplements (twenty-two is not that many really). What I want to discuss
right now, though, is the connection that stress has to hair loss. As you
know, genetics as well as severe, life threatening illnesses and their
chemically active treatments are major factors to—or causes of— hair
loss. What about stress? Does that old saying mean much? You know,
"Don't worry so much dear, or you'll lose all your hair."

Research has found that a certain level of constant, ongoing stress
affects our health in many negative ways, and one of these ways is,
unfortunately, hair loss. Of course, there are stressful situations and
events in every person's life. That's life—a series of ups and downs, like
a roller coaster at times. You still want to try, though, to level this roller
coaster as much as possible, not just to help thwart stress-related hair
loss but also to keep your immune system functioning at an optimum
level. You need to keep yourself in that sweet state of homeostasis,
which means balance.

There is the subject of *metabolic* balance, which is achieved through
proper nutrition after going through metabolic testing. There is also
physical and chemical balance, and there is the kind of balance that I
am focusing on here, a person's regular *mental* and *emotional* state of
mind. In life sh-t happens, but you can help lessen the impact when a
negative, life-changing event comes your way, or even dull the more
common daily stressors that come along in life at any given moment.
To do this you must gain a sense of control and purpose in your everyday routine. You must work at eliminating any constant, unnecessary
stress. Notice I used the word "everyday." That is because *consistency*
is key. Consistency is vital for this to work. You need to consistently eat
right, regularly exercise, and interact socially with others, on a regular
basis, with whom you feel a real connection and those who leave you
with a good feeling after you spend time with them.

Practice regular breathing exercises. Take up interesting hobbies
that keep you from sitting around and thinking too much. Try to find

joy in whatever it is you do for a living if you don't already love your job, or change careers if you can. Sometimes just putting in the effort and having the sheer will to live a more balanced life and to be happier is enough to make you happy and, as a result, lose less hair.

Fall in Love Already!

Please do not laugh. I really mean what I am going to say here. This may sound a little corny, but I don't feel that I am going out on a limb when I suggest this. The emotional benefit you get by simply falling in love with, or even having a little crush on, someone is so powerful that it actually can propel your immune system into overdrive, giving it the boost it may need at any given time. Doesn't sound so ridiculous after all, does it?

The effect on the immune system, I believe, from this feeling of love or infatuation can be sometimes unmatched by even the most powerful of nutritional foods and supplements. The emotional state of falling in love can help the immune system fight off unwanted viruses, bacteria, free radicals, and even precancerous cells through your body's inherent mind-body connection, thereby enabling you to live a longer, healthier life. It is said that married couples live longer than single people. Now, being happily divorced and single myself, I am on the fence with this one. I do believe that happiness is key. I am not so sure that being married equates to being happy. What I am pretty sure about, however, is that as you grow into older age, you will probably be happier and healthier to be part of a unit or a married couple, which I myself look forward to.

Now back to that special feeling of romantic love, which leaves one with an invigorating high felt sometimes on an even subconscious level. It's highly motivating, isn't it? This feeling makes a person want to better themselves almost immediately, providing a newly found sense of internal energy that makes him or her *want* to exercise, eat better, and actively start anew. As a result he or she starts to look better and, more important, *feel* better.

No matter how old you are, just acquiring a simple crush on someone is enough to pull you out of a rut. If you aren't single but aren't in that intoxicating state of new, romantic bliss either, try to find a way to fall in love again with your significant other. The emotional rewards and health benefits will be well worth it in the long run, and isn't that what this book is about? Longevity?

Okay, that is all I have for now. (The nutritional discoveries made by scientists and researchers never stop.) I hope that by reading my book you have gained the will to improve and gain control over your health, and feel better equipped with the ammunition needed to combat premature aging. Don't just roll over—fight! Kick aging to the curb! Those body-invading, disease-causing, cell-changing, wrinkle-forming oxidants and toxins don't stand a chance against a well-informed, butt-kicking soldier like you.

REFERENCES

Books

Jean Carper, *Food: Your Miracle Medicine* (New York: HarperCollins Publishers, 1993).

Jeffrey Dover, M.D., and Cara Birnbaum, *The Youth Equation: Take 10 Years off Your Face* (Hoboken, New Jersey: John Wiley & Sons, 2009).

Rory Freedman and Kim Barnouin, *Skinny Bitch* (Philadelphia: Running Press, 2005).

Carla Krupp, *How Not to Look Old: Fast and Effortless Ways to Look 10 Years Younger, 10 Pounds Lighter, 10 Times Better* (New York: Stonesong Press, 2008).

Kathleen L. Mahan, MS, RD, CDE, and Sylvia Escott-Stump, MA, RD, *Krause's Food, Nutrition and Diet Therapy, Ninth Edition* (Philadelphia: W.B. Saunders Company, 1996).

C. Norman Shealy, M.D., *The Complete Family Guide to Alternative Medicine: An Illustrated Encyclopedia of Natural Healing* (Rockport, Massachusetts: Element Books, 1996).

Dr. Andrew Stanway, M.B., M.R.C.P., and Richard Grossman PhD, *The New Natural Family Doctor: The Authoritative Self-Help Guide to Health and Natural Medicine* (London: Gaia Books Ltd., 1987).

Andrew Weil, M.D. *Spontaneous Healing: How to Discover and Embrace Your Body's Natural Ability to Maintain and Heal Itself* (New York: A. Knopf, 1995).

Bradley J. Willcox; Craig D Willcox, PhD; and Suzuki, Makoto, M.D., *The Okinawa Diet Plan: Get Leaner, Live Longer, and Never Feel Hungry* (New York: Three Rivers Press, 2005).

Tom Williams, PhD, *Chinese Medicine* (New York: Barnes & Noble Books, 1996).

Articles

Aleta Capelle, "Exercise for Your Heart," *Mayo Clinic Health Letter,* Vol. 29, 2:1 (Feb. 2011).

Aleta Capelle, "Telomeres and Health," *Mayo Clinic Health Letter,* Vol. 29, 3:7 (March 2011).

Robert Capelli and Gerald R. Cysewski, PhD, "The Neuroprotective Effect of Astaxanthin" *Dynamic Chiropractic Nutritional Wellness,* Vol. 6, 1 (Feb. 2010).

"Benefits of Curcumin," http://www.curcumin.net/health-remedies 2009.

D. Dye, "Apple Polyphenols Extend Lifespan in Fruit Fly Experiment," *Life Extension* (June 2011): 15.

D. Dye, "Coffee Drinking Linked with Lower Risk of Endometrial Cancer," *Life Extension* (Nov. 2011): 23.

Carley Eder, "The Awesome Apple," *Life Extension* (July 2011): 85–87.

J. Finkle, "Milestone Study to Look at Genetic Effects of Caloric Restriction," *Life Extension* (June 2011): 15.

Michelle Flagg, "Link Between Alcohol and Cancer Death," *Life Extension* (Dec. 2011): 59–66.

Alan H. Goodman, PhD., "Why Genes Don't Count (for Racial Differences in Health)," *American Journal of Public Health* 90 (2000): 1699–1702.

Knut Holt, "The Benefits, Joys, and Danger of the Sunlight," http://www.healthguidance.org.

Dr. Ronald Klatz and Dr. Robert Goldman, "Age Is Just a Number," *To Your Health* (Dec. 2009): 14–17.

Dr. Ronald Klatz and Dr. Robert Goldman, "Why Gamble on Your Health? 7 Ways to Reduce Your Cancer Risk," *To Your Health* (Feb. 2010): 22.

Simin Liu, M.D., ScD, "A Prospective Study of Whole-Grain Intake and Risk of Type 2 Diabetes Mellitus in US Women," *American Journal of Public Health* 90 (2000): 1409–1415.

April May Maple, "The Effect of Weather on Mental Health," http://www.helium.com, March 2009.

Paul Meglothin and Meredith Averill, "Success Stories: Real People Who Have Changed Their Lives by Altering Caloric Intake," *Life Extension* (Dec. 2011): 71–77.

Kara Michaels, "Halt Sugar-Induced Cell Aging," *Life Extension* (Jan. 2012): 59–65.

"New Study Validates Hair Growth Mechanism of Resveratrol/Curcumin," http://www.hairloss-research.org, July 2011.

Gail Richardson, "Beyond Eye Health: How Astaxanthin Combats Degenerative Disease," *Life Extension*, (July 2011): 55–62.

Irwin H. Rosenburg, M.D., "Now, Bottled Water With Vitamins and Herbs," *Tufts University Health & Nutrition Letter*, Vol. 20, 5:1 (2002).

Dr. David Ryan, "You Need Your Sleep," *To Your Health* (Dec. 2009): 19–21.

Elizabeth Scott M.S., "Stress and Hair Loss: What Are the Causes of Hair Loss?" http://stress.about.com, May 14, 2011.

Dr. David Seaman, "Year-Round Skin Protection," *To Your Health* (Jan. 2011): 10–13.

S. Sharma, K. Chopra, S.K. Kulkarni, and J.N. Agrewala, "Resveratrol and Curcumin Suppress Immune Response Through CD28/CTLA-4 and CD80 Co-Stimulatory Pathway," *Clinical and Experimental Immunology of Translational Immunology,* Vol. 147, 1 (2007).

Alex Vasquez, DC, ND; Gilbert Manson, M.D.; and John Cannell, M.D.: "The Clinical Importance of Vitamin D (Cholecalciferol): A Paradigm Shift With Implications for All Healthcare Providers," *Continuing Medical Education. Alternative Therapies*, Vol. 10:5 (2004).